MW00781896

Introduction 5

Guidelines for Using
  the Food Exchanges 7

    The Food Guide Pyramid 9
    Choosing a Calorie Level 11
    Calorie Level Exchanges 13
    Using Food Exchanges 15

Food Exchanges 21

Fast-Food Restaurant Healthy Choices 47

FIRST PLACE

FOOD
EXCHANGE

POCKET GUIDE

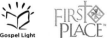

Gospel Light is an evangelical Christian publisher dedicated to serving the local church. We believe God's vision for Gospel Light is to provide church leaders with biblical, user-friendly materials that will help them evangelize, disciple and minister to children, youth and families.

It is our prayer that this Gospel Light resource will help you discover biblical truth for your own life and help you minister to others. May God richly bless you.

For a free catalog of resources from Gospel Light, please call your Christian supplier or contact us at 1-800-4-GOSPEL or www.gospellight.com.

PUBLISHING STAFF
William T. Greig, Chairman
Kyle Duncan, Publisher
Dr. Elmer L. Towns, Senior Consulting Publisher
Pam Weston, Senior Editor
Patti Pennington Virtue, Associate Editor
Hilary Young, Editorial Assistant
Jessie Minassian, Editorial Assistant
Bayard Taylor, M.Div., Senior Editor, Biblical and Theological Issues
Samantha A. Hsu, Cover and Internal Designer

ISBN 0-8307-3232-2
© 2003 First Place
All rights reserved.
Printed in the U.S.A.

Any omission of credits is unintentional. The publisher requests documentation for future printings.

CAUTION
The information contained in this book is intended to be solely informational and educational. It is assumed that the First Place participant will consult a medical or health professional before beginning First Place or any other weight-loss or physical-fitness program.

INTRODUCTION

The First Place program was developed over 20 years ago as the result of a godly desire placed in the hearts of a group of Christians to establish a Christ-centered weight control program. What began as a Christ-centered weight-loss program has evolved into a nationally recognized total-health program. Today the First Place program is used in every state and many foreign countries. Thousands of lives have been changed.

Matthew 6:33: "Seek first his kingdom and his righteousness, and all these things will be given to you as well" was chosen as the theme verse for the program. Hence, the name First Place.

The First Place program addresses all areas of a person's life—spiritual, mental, emotional and physical—and it includes Bible study, small-group support, accountability, a proven com-monsense nutrition plan, exercise, record keeping and Scripture memory.

This *Food Exchange Pocket Guide* is based on the First Place Live-It plan as described in the First Place *Member's Guide* on pages 31 to 73. However, unlike the listing by food group in the *Member's Guide*, the exchanges listed in this book are arranged in easy-to-find alphabetical order. You will also find included in this handy resource the basic information needed to understand the food exchanges and apply them to your individual needs. Additional information can be found in the *Member's Guide*. Also provided is a listing of the healthiest choices at the most popular fast-food restaurants.

May this handy little book help guide you to a healthier, more fulfilling life.

GUIDELINES FOR USING THE FOOD EXCHANGES

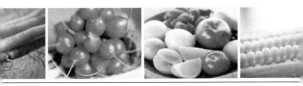

THE FOOD GUIDE PYRAMID*

For everything God created is good.
1 Timothy 4:4

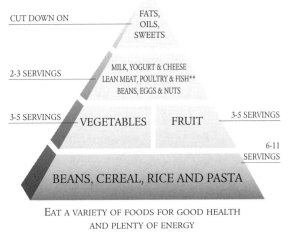

CUT DOWN ON — FATS, OILS, SWEETS

2-3 SERVINGS — MILK, YOGURT & CHEESE
LEAN MEAT, POULTRY & FISH**
BEANS, EGGS & NUTS

3-5 SERVINGS — VEGETABLES | FRUIT — 3-5 SERVINGS

6-11 SERVINGS

BEANS, CEREAL, RICE AND PASTA

EAT A VARIETY OF FOODS FOR GOOD HEALTH
AND PLENTY OF ENERGY

The Food Guide Pyramid, introduced in 1992 by the United States Department of Agriculture (USDA) and now adapted by most major health and nutrition organizations, offers a visual and practical way to put healthy nutrition into practice. The pyramid divides all foods into five groups based on their nutritional similarities and the number of servings needed for a healthy diet (much like exchanges). It includes an additional category for fats, oils and sweets, which should be eaten sparingly. Each food group supplies some, but not all, of the nutrients you need. No one food or food group is more important than another; you need them all for nutritional health. By eating a variety of foods from each group, sticking with the recommended number of daily servings and putting into practice the principles of portion control, the pyramid and the Live-It plan will help you achieve your goals for healthy weight and good health.

Adapted from United States Department of Agriculture
Food Guide Pyramid

*The Food Guide Pyramid has been adapted by First Place to more closely reflect our program and recommendations.

**Note: A serving of meat, poultry or fish is two to three ounces, compared to one-ounce servings for the exchange list.

CHOOSING A CALORIE LEVEL

The following tables are designed to help you choose a daily calorie level for healthy weight loss. Choose the recommended calorie level for your age and body weight. (**Note:** See pages 34-35 in the First Place *Member's Guide* for more information on finding your healthy weight.) This calorie level is your starting point for the Live-It food exchange plan.

RECOMMENDED CALORIE RANGES FOR WOMEN					
Age↓/Weight→	100-119	120-139	140-159	160-179	180+
20-39	1400	1400	1500	1600	1600
40-59	1200	1400	1400	1500	1500
60+	1200	1200	1400	1400	1400

Note: If your goal is to maintain weight, add 300-500 calories to your plan.

RECOMMENDED CALORIE RANGES FOR MEN					
Age↓/Weight→	140-159	160-179	180-199	200-219	220+
20-39	1800	1800	2000	2200	2400
40-59	1600	1800	1800	2000	2200
60+	1500	1600	1800	1800	2000

Note: If your goal is to maintain weight, add 400-600 calories to your plan.

These tables use the best available methods for estimating a calorie level for healthy weight loss; however, your needs may be different. Age, gender, heredity, body size and physical activity influence the number of calories your body needs. It's best to lose weight at a rate of one-half to two pounds each week. Adjust the calorie plan up or down based on how you feel and how well you are meeting your goals. If you are losing more than two pounds a week, change to the next higher calorie level. Also, if you're not losing weight, check your portion sizes—many people don't realize how much they're eating!

CALORIE LEVEL EXCHANGES

This daily exchange plan allows you to personalize your Live-It plan based on your nutritional needs and eating preferences. Choosing the lowest number of exchanges from each food group will give you fewer calories than listed. To stay within your calorie level, don't choose the higher number of exchanges from more than one food group. You can, however, choose the highest number of exchanges for the fruit and vegetable groups.

DAILY EXCHANGE PLANS						
Calorie Levels	Bread/ Starch	Vegetable	Fruit	Meat	Milk	Fat
1200	5-6	3	2-3	4-5	2-3	3-4
1400	6-7	3-4	3-4	5-6	2-3	3-4
1500	7-8	3-4	3-4	5-6	2-3	3-4
1600	8-9	3-4	3-4	6-7	2-3	3-4
1800	10-11	3-4	3-4	6-7	2-3	4-5
2000	11-12	4-5	4-5	6-7	2-3	5-6
2200	12-13	4-5	4-5	7-8	2-3	6-7
2400	13-14	4-5	4-5	8-9	2-3	7-8
2600	14-15	5	5	9-10	2-3	7-8
2800	15-16	5	5	9-10	2-3	9-10

Note: The food exchanges break down to approximately 50-55% carbohydrate, 15-20% protein and 25-30% fat.

Designing Your Personal Eating Plan

For your personalized eating plan, take the following steps:

- Choose your appropriate daily calorie level from the Choosing a Calorie Level table (p. 11).
- Choose your daily exchange allowance from the Daily Exchange Plans chart on previous page.
- From your daily exchange allowance, record the total exchanges for each food group in the following My Live-It plan chart.
- Distribute your daily exchange allowances into the three time periods in your plan.

Here is a sample plan:

My Live-It Plan = __1600__ Calories				
	Exchanges			
	Morning	Midday	Evening	Totals
Breads/Starches	2	3	4	9
Vegetables		1	2	3
Fruits	1	1	1	3
Meat	2	2	2	6
Milk	1	$\frac{1}{2}$	$\frac{1}{2}$	2
Fat	1	1	1	3

My Live-It Plan = _____ Calories				
	Exchanges			
	Morning	Midday	Evening	Totals
Breads/Starches				
Vegetables				
Fruits				
Meat				
Milk				
Fat				

USING FOOD EXCHANGES

Foods are divided into seven exchange lists: bread/starch, meat, vegetable, fruit, milk, fat and free foods. All the foods within a food list contain approximately the same amount of nutrients and calories per serving, which means that one serving of a food from the bread list may be exchanged (or substituted) for one serving of any other item in the bread list.

The seven exchange lists, or food groups, were developed to aid in menu planning. The individual diet plan prescribed by a physician and/or registered dietitian indicates the number of servings from each food group that should be eaten at each meal and snack. The following chart shows the amount of nutrients and number of calories in one serving from each food group. If you cannot, or choose not to, eat from a particular food group, consult with a physician or nutritionist to ensure proper nutrition.

	Carbo-hydrates (in grams)	Protein (in grams)	Fat (in grams)	Calories
Bread/Starch	15	3	trace	80
Meat				
Lean	–	7	3	55
Medium Fat	–	7	5	75
High Fat	–	7	8	100
Vegetable	5	2	–	25
Fruit	15	–	–	60
Milk				
Fat Free	12	8	trace	90
Very Low Fat	12	8	3	105
Low Fat	12	8	5	120
Whole	12	8	8	150

Bread/Starch Exchanges

Each item on the bread/starch exchange list contains approximately **15 grams of carbohydrates, 3 grams of protein, a trace of fat and 80 calories**. The foods in this versatile list contain similar amounts of nutrients. The bread/starch list encompasses cereals, crackers, dried beans, starchy vegetables, breads and prepared foods.

Meat Exchanges

Each item on the meat exchange list contains approximately **7 grams of protein, some fat and no carbohydrates**. The meat exchange is divided into three groups according to how much fat it contains and **calories per serving will vary** accordingly.

Vegetable Exchanges

Each item on the vegetable exchange list contains **5 grams of carbohydrates and 2 grams of protein, for a total of 25 calories**. The generous use of assorted nutritious vegetables in your diet contributes to sound health and vitality. Enjoy them cooked or raw.

Fruit Exchanges

Each item on the fruit list contains **15 grams of carbohydrates and 60 calories**. Fruits are a wonderful addition to your food plan because of their complex carbohydrates, dietary fiber and other food components linked to good health. They are also readily available, taste great and are quick and easy to prepare.

Milk Exchanges

Each item on the milk exchange list contains **12 grams of carbohydrates, 8 grams of protein and 90 calories. Fat content and calories vary** depending on the product you use. As a general rule, milk exchanges can be divided into four main categories, which are outlined in the food exchanges list.

Fat Exchanges

Each item on the fat exchange list contains **5 grams of fat and 45 calories**. The Live-It plan limits your fat intake to 25 percent of your daily calorie total. One-half of your fat allotment comes from your lean meat choices. The other half is chosen from the fat exchange list.

Free Foods

The items on the free foods exchange list are foods very low in nutritional value and usually low in calories. Limit the total number of calories from this exchange to 50 per day.

DON'T FORGET WATER

- For good health, drink at least eight 8-ounce glasses of water a day. For every 25 pounds over your healthy weight, add an additional 8 ounces of water.
- Thirst is not always the best indication of the body's need for water. Plan to drink water regularly to avoid dehydration.
- Adequate water is necessary to burn fat.
- Water helps to maintain proper muscle tone by giving muscles their natural ability to contract. It also helps to prevent sagging skin.
- Water can help relieve constipation.
- If drinking eight glasses of water seems impossible, start at your own pace and increase as you can until you reach the recommended amount.

FOOD EXCHANGES

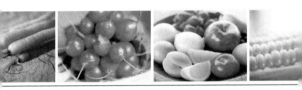

Item	Amount	Exchanges
Alfalfa sprouts	1 c.	FREE ^
All-Bran cereal	½ c.	1 bread
Almond butter	1 tsp.	1 fat
Almonds, dry-roasted	6 whole	1 fat
Animal crackers, low-fat, low-sugar	1 oz.	1 bread + ½ fat
Apple	1 medium (4 oz.)	1 fruit
Apple juice	½ c.	1 fruit
Apples, dried	4 rings (¾ oz.)	1 fruit
Applesauce, unsweetened	½ c.	1 fruit
Apricots, canned	½ c. (4 oz.)	1 fruit
Apricots, dried	7 halves (¾ oz.)	1 fruit
Apricots, raw	4 medium	1 fruit
Artichoke, cooked	½ c.	1 vegetable
Artichoke, raw	1 c.	1 vegetable
Asparagus, cooked	½ c.	1 vegetable
Asparagus, raw	1 c.	1 vegetable
Avocado	⅛ medium	1 fat

* Foods with this symbol are high in saturated fat and are not recommended.
^ Daily total for FREE foods with this symbol should not exceed 50 calories.

	Item	Amount	Exchanges
B	Bacon bits, imitation	∧	FREE
	Bacon grease	1 tsp.*	1 fat
	Bacon, pork	1 slice*	1 fat
	Bacon, turkey	2 slices	1 meat + ½ fat
	Bagel	½ (1 oz.)	1 bread
	Bamboo shoots, cooked	½ c.	1 vegetable
	Bamboo shoots, raw	1 c.	1 vegetable
	Banana	½ (3 oz.)	1 fruit
	Barbecue sauce	¼ c.	1 bread
	Barbecue sauce (as condiment)	∧	FREE
	Barley, cooked	⅓ c.	1 bread
	Barley, dry	1½ tbsp.	1 bread
	Bean sprouts, cooked	½ c.	1 vegetable
	Bean sprouts, raw	1 c.	1 vegetable
	Beans, baked	¼ c.	1 bread
	Beans (green, Italian, wax), cooked	½ c.	1 vegetable
	Beans (kidney, pinto, white), cooked	1 c.	2 bread + 1 lean meat
	Beans (kidney, pinto, white), cooked	⅓ c.	1 bread
	Beans, lima	½ c.	1 bread
	Beans, refried	⅓ c.	1 bread + ½ fat

* Foods with this symbol are high in saturated fat and are not recommended.
∧ Daily total for FREE foods with this symbol should not exceed 50 calories.

Item	Amount	Exchanges
Beans, refried, fat-free	⅓ c.	1 bread
Beef, high-fat (prime cuts such as brisket, corned beef and ribs)	1 oz.	1 meat + 1 fat
Beef, lean (breakfast steak, filet mignon, flank steak, lean ground beef, London broil, pot roast, sirloin, strip steak, tenderloin, top round)	1 oz.	1 meat
Beef, medium-fat (chuck roast, cubed steak, ground beef, Porterhouse steak, rib roast, rump roast, T-bone)	1 oz.	1 meat + ½ fat
Beets	½ c.	1 vegetable
Biscuit	1 medium (2½ in.)	1 bread + 1 fat
Blackberries, raw	¾ c.	1 fruit
Blueberries, raw	¾ c.	1 fruit
Bok choy	1 c.	FREE
Bologna	1 oz.	1 meat + 1 fat
Bouillon	^	FREE
Boysenberries	¾ c.	1 fruit
Bran cereal, concentrated	⅓ c.	1 bread
Bran cereal, flaked	½ c.	1 bread
Bran, raw, unprocessed	½ c.	1 bread
Bratwurst	1 oz.	1 meat + 1 fat

* Foods with this symbol are high in saturated fat and are not recommended.
^ Daily total for FREE foods with this symbol should not exceed 50 calories.

Item	Amount	Exchanges
Bread crumbs, dried	2 tbsp.	1 bread
Bread, diet (40 calories per slice)	2 slices	1 bread
Bread, pumpernickel	1 slice (1 oz.)	1 bread
Bread, rye	1 slice (1 oz.)	1 bread
Bread, whole-wheat, white, French, Italian	1 slice (1 oz.)	1 bread
Breadsticks, crisp (4x1 1/2-in.)	2 ($\frac{2}{3}$ oz.)	1 bread
Broccoli, cooked	$\frac{1}{2}$ c.	1 vegetable
Broccoli, raw	1 c.	1 vegetable
Broth	^	FREE
Bulgur, cooked	$\frac{1}{2}$ c.	1 bread
Bun, hamburger or hot dog	$\frac{1}{2}$ (1 oz.)	1 bread
Butter	1 tsp.*	1 fat
Butter flavoring, powdered	^	FREE
Butter, reduced-fat	1 tbsp.*	1 fat
Buttermilk, fat-free	1 c.	1 milk

* Foods with this symbol are high in saturated fat and are not recommended.
^ Daily total for FREE foods with this symbol should not exceed 50 calories.

Item	Amount	Exchanges
Cabbage, cooked	½ c.	1 vegetable
Cabbage, Chinese	1 c.	FREE
Cabbage, raw	1 c.	FREE
Canadian bacon	1 oz.	1 meat
Candies, sugar-free	^	FREE
Cantaloupe	⅓ melon (7 oz.) or 1 c. cubed	1 fruit
Carambola (starfruit)	3 (7½ oz.)	1 fruit
Carbonated sugar-free soda	^	FREE
Carbonated water	^	FREE
Carrot juice	½ c.	1 vegetable
Cashews, dry-roasted	1 tbsp.	1 fat
Catsup	¼ c.	1 bread
Catsup, as condiment	^	FREE
Celery	1 c.	FREE
Cereal, 100% bran	⅓ c.	1 bread
Cereals, cooked	½ c.	1 bread
Cereals, ready-to-eat, unsweetened	¾ c.	1 bread
Cheerios	¾ c.	1 bread
Cheese	2 oz.	1 milk
Cheese (all regular cheeses such as American, blue, cheddar, Colby, Monterey Jack and Swiss)	1 oz.	1 meat + 1 fat

C

* Foods with this symbol are high in saturated fat and are not recommended.
^ Daily total for FREE foods with this symbol should not exceed 50 calories.

Item	Amount	Exchanges
Cheese, fat-free	1 oz.	1 meat
Cheese (light, skim or part-skim milk cheeses)	1 oz.	1 meat + ½ fat
Cheese, Parmesan, grated	2 tbsp.	1 meat
Cheese spread	1 tbsp.*	1 fat
Cherries, canned	½ c.	1 fruit
Cherries, raw	12 large (3½ oz.)	1 fruit
Chewing gum, sugar-free	∧	FREE
Chicken, baked	1 oz.	1 meat + 1 fat
Chicken fat	1 tsp.*	1 fat
Chicken, fried	1 oz.	1 meat + 1 fat
Chicken noodle soup, canned	1 c.	½ bread + ½ fat
Chili sauce	¼ c.	1 bread
Chili sauce (as condiment)	∧	FREE
Chips, corn	1 oz.	1 bread + 2 fats
Chips, potato	1 oz.	1 bread + 2 fats
Chips, tortilla	5	1 bread
Chitterlings	½ oz.*	1 fat
Chocolate, baking	1 oz.	1 bread + 2 fats

* Foods with this symbol are high in saturated fat and are not recommended.
∧ Daily total for FREE foods with this symbol should not exceed 50 calories.

Item	Amount	Exchanges
Chocolate, unsweetened	1 oz.*	1 bread + 2 fats
Chocolate-milk mix, sugar-free	^	FREE
Chow mein noodles	½ c.	1 bread + 1 fat
Cilantro	1 c.	FREE
Club soda	^	FREE
Cocktail sauce	^	FREE
Cocoa	5 tbsp.	1 bread
Cocoa powder, unsweetened	^	FREE
Coconut, shredded	2 tbsp.*	1 fat
Coffee	^	FREE
Coffee whitener, liquid	2 tbsp.*	1 fat
Coffee whitener, powder	4 tsp.*	1 fat
Coffee whiteners, nondairy	^	FREE
Cooking spray	^	FREE
Corn	½ c.	1 bread
Cornbread (2-inch cube)	1 2 oz.	1 bread + 1 fat
Cornflakes	¾ c.	1 bread
Cornish game hen	1 oz.	1 meat
Cornmeal	2½ tbsp.	1 bread
Corn-on-the-cob	1 6-in. ear	1 bread
Cornstarch	2 tbsp.	1 bread
Cottage cheese	¼ c.	1 meat

* Foods with this symbol are high in saturated fat and are not recommended.
^ Daily total for FREE foods with this symbol should not exceed 50 calories.

Item	Amount	Exchanges
Cottage cheese	½ c.	1 milk
Couscous, cooked	⅓ c.	1 bread
Crab apples	¾ c. (2¾ oz.)	1 fruit
Cracker, round butter-type	6	1 bread + 1 fat
Cracker, saltine	6	1 bread
Cranberry juice	⅓ c.	1 fruit
Cream cheese	1 tbsp.*	1 fat
Cream cheese, fat-free	2 oz.	1 meat
Cream cheese, light	2 tbsp.*	1 fat
Cream, half-and-half	2 tbsp.*	1 fat
Cream of broccoli soup, canned	½ c.	1 bread
Cream of celery soup, canned	½ c.	1 bread
Cream of chicken soup, canned	½ c.	1 bread + 1 fat
Cream of mushroom soup, canned	½ c.	½ bread + ½ fat
Cress, garden	1 c.	FREE
Croissant	1 small	1 bread + 2 fats
Croutons, low-fat	1 c.	1 bread
Cucumber	1 c.	FREE

* Foods with this symbol are high in saturated fat and are not recommended.
⌐ Daily total for FREE foods with this symbol should not exceed 50 calories.

Item	Amount	Exchanges	
Date, dried	2½ medium	1 fruit	**D**
Dewberries	¾ c. (3 oz.)	1 fruit	
Drink mixes, sugar-free	^	FREE	
Dry nonfat milk	¼ c.	1 milk	
Duck	1 oz.	1 meat + ½ fat	
Egg	1	1 meat + ½ fat	**E**
Egg substitutes	¼ c.	1 meat	
Egg whites	3	1 meat	
Eggplant, cooked	½ c.	1 vegetable	
Eggplant, raw	1 c.	1 vegetable	
Enchilada sauce	^	FREE	
Endive	1 c.	FREE	
English muffin	½	1 bread	
Escarole	1 c.	FREE	
Evaporated skim milk	½ c.	1 milk	
Evaporated whole milk	½ c.	1 milk + 2 fats	

* Foods with this symbol are high in saturated fat and are not recommended.
^ Daily total for FREE foods with this symbol should not exceed 50 calories.

	Item	Amount	Exchanges
F	Fiber One cereal	⅔ c.	1 bread
	Figs, dried	1½	1 fruit
	Figs, raw (2 inches)	2	1 fruit
	Fish (canned tuna in oil and canned salmon)	¼ c.	1 meat + ½ fat
	Fish (catfish, haddock, halibut, herring, orange roughy, trout, salmon or tuna in water), baked	1 oz.	1 meat
	Fish, fried	1 oz.	1 meat + 1 fat
	Flour, soybean	½ c.	1 bread + 2 meats + 1 fat
	Flour, white or whole-wheat	1 c.	5 breads
	Frankfurter, low-fat	1 oz.	1 meat
	Frankfurter, (up to 5 grams fat/oz.)	1 oz.	1 meat + ½ fat
	Frankfurter, (up to 8 grams of fat/oz.)	1 oz.	1 meat + 1 fat
	French fries (2 to 3½ in. long)	10 fries	1 bread + 1 fat
	Fruit cocktail, canned	½ c.	1 fruit
	Fruit spreads, sugar-free	^	FREE

* Foods with this symbol are high in saturated fat and are not recommended.
^ Daily total for FREE foods with this symbol should not exceed 50 calories.

Item	Amount	Exchanges
Game (venison, rabbit)	1 oz.	1 meat
Gelatin, sugar-free	^	FREE
Goose	1 oz.	1 meat + $\frac{1}{2}$ fat
Gooseberries	1 c. (5 oz.)	1 fruit
Graham crackers	3 2-inch squares	1 bread
Grape juice	$\frac{1}{3}$ c.	1 fruit
Grapefruit	$\frac{1}{2}$ grapefruit	1 fruit
Grapefruit juice	$\frac{1}{2}$ c.	1 fruit
Grapefruit, segments	$\frac{3}{4}$ c.	1 fruit
Grape-Nuts flakes	$\frac{1}{2}$ c.	1 bread
Grape-Nuts nuggets	3 tbsp.	1 bread
Grapes	17 small	1 fruit
Gravy, home-style	$\frac{1}{4}$ c.*	1 fat
Gravy, packaged	$\frac{1}{2}$ c.*	1 fat
Green onion	1 c.	FREE
Grits, cooked	$\frac{1}{2}$ c.	1 bread
Ground pork	1 oz.	1 meat + 1 fat
Ground turkey	1 oz.	1 meat + $\frac{1}{2}$ fat

G

* Foods with this symbol are high in saturated fat and are not recommended.
^ Daily total for FREE foods with this symbol should not exceed 50 calories.

	Item	Amount	Exchanges
H	Ham	1 oz.	1 meat
	Heart	1 oz.	1 meat + $\frac{1}{2}$ fat
	Hearts of palm, cooked	$\frac{1}{2}$ c.	1 vegetable
	Hearts of palm, raw	1 c.	1 vegetable
	Hominy	$\frac{1}{2}$ c.	1 bread
	Honeydew melon, cubed	1 c.	1 fruit
	Honeydew melon, sliced	$\frac{1}{8}$ melon	1 fruit
	Horseradish	^	FREE
	Hot chocolate, sugar-free	1 packet	$\frac{1}{2}$ milk
	Hot peppers	1 c.	FREE
	Hummus	$\frac{1}{4}$ c.	1 bread + 1 fat
I	Ice cream, sugar-free, fat-free	3 oz.	1 bread
	Ice-cream bar, sugar-free	^	FREE
	Iced tea, sugar-free	^	FREE
J	Jicama, cooked	$\frac{1}{2}$ c.	1 vegetable
	Jicama, raw	1 c.	1 vegetable

* Foods with this symbol are high in saturated fat and are not recommended.
^ Daily total for FREE foods with this symbol should not exceed 50 calories.

Item	Amount	Exchanges	
Kale, cooked	½ c.	1 vegetable	**K**
Kale, raw	1 c.	1 vegetable	
Kasha, cooked	½ c.	1 bread	
Kidney	1 oz.	1 meat + ½ fat	
Kiwi	1 large (3¼ oz.)	1 fruit	
Knockwurst	1 oz.	1 meat + 1 fat	
Kohlrabi, cooked	½ c.	1 vegetable	
Kohlrabi, raw	1 c.	1 vegetable	
Lactaid	1 c.	1 milk	**L**
Lamb (chops, leg and roast)	1 oz.	1 meat + ½ fat	
Lamb, ground	1 oz.	1 meat + 1 fat	
Lard	1 tsp.*	1 fat	
Leeks, cooked	½ c.	1 vegetable	
Leeks, raw	½ c.	1 vegetable	
Lemon juice	1 c.	1 fruit	
Lemon juice, as seasoning	^	FREE	
Lentils	⅓ c.	1 bread	
Lentils	1 c.	2 bread + 1 lean meat	
Lettuce	1 c.	FREE	

* Foods with this symbol are high in saturated fat and are not recommended.
^ Daily total for FREE foods with this symbol should not exceed 50 calories.

Item	Amount	Exchanges
Lime juice	1 c.	1 fruit
Lime juice, as seasoning	^	FREE
Liver	1 oz.	1 meat + ½ fat
Luncheon meat, fat-free	1 oz.	1 meat
Luncheon meat, high fat (bologna, salami, pimento loaf)	1 oz.	1 meat + 1 fat
Luncheon meat, lean (up to 5 grams of fat)	1 oz.	1 meat + ½ fat
Malt (dry)	1 tbsp.	1 bread
Mandarin oranges, canned in own juice	¾ c.	1 fruit
Mango	½ mango (3 oz.)	1 fruit
Margarine	1 tsp.	1 fat
Margarine, light	1 tbsp.	1 fat
Matzo	¾ oz.	1 bread
Mayonnaise	1 tsp.	1 fat
Mayonnaise, fat-free	^	FREE
Mayonnaise, light	1 tbsp.	1 fat
Meat fat	1 tsp.*	1 fat
Melba toast	5 slices	1 bread
Milk, 1½% or 2%	1 c.	1 milk + 1 fat
Milk, 1%	1 c.	1 milk + ½ fat

M

* Foods with this symbol are high in saturated fat and are not recommended.
^ Daily total for FREE foods with this symbol should not exceed 50 calories.

Item	Amount	Exchanges
Milk, nonfat or $\frac{1}{2}$%	1 c.	1 milk
Milk, whole	1 c.	1 milk + 2 fats
Millet, cooked	$\frac{1}{4}$ c.	1 bread
Miso	$\frac{1}{2}$ c.	1 bread + 2 meats + 1 fat
Muffin, plain, small	1	1 bread + 1 fat
Mulberries	1 c. (5 oz.)	1 fruit
Mushrooms, cooked	$\frac{1}{2}$ c.	1 vegetable
Mushrooms, raw	1 c.	FREE
Mustard	^	FREE
Nectarine	1 medium (5 oz.)	1 fruit
Nuts, chopped (almonds, pecans, walnuts)	1 tbsp.	1 fat

N

* Foods with this symbol are high in saturated fat and are not recommended.
^ Daily total for FREE foods with this symbol should not exceed 50 calories.

	Item	Amount	Exchanges
O	Oil (corn, cottonseed, olive, peanut, safflower, soybean and sunflower)	1 tsp.	1 fat
	Okra	1 c.	1 vegetable
	Onions, cooked	½ c.	1 vegetable
	Onions, raw	1 c.	1 vegetable
	Orange	1 medium (6½ oz.)	1 fruit
	Orange juice	½ c.	1 fruit
	Orange juice concentrate	2 tbsp. (1 oz.)	1 fruit
	Oyster crackers	24	1 bread
P	Pancake	2 4-in.	1 bread + 1 fat
	Papaya	1 c. (8 oz.)	1 fruit
	Parsley	1 c.	FREE
	Passion fruit	4 4 oz.	1 fruit
	Pasta, cooked	½ c.	1 bread
	Pea pods	½ c.	1 vegetable
	Peaches	1 peach or ¾ c.	1 fruit
	Peaches, canned	½ c. or 2 halves	1 fruit
	Peanut butter, low-fat or regular	1 tsp.	1 fat
	Peanut butter, low-fat or regular	1 tbsp.	1 meat + 1 fat

* Foods with this symbol are high in saturated fat and are not recommended.
^ Daily total for FREE foods with this symbol should not exceed 50 calories.

Item	Amount	Exchanges
Peanuts	20 small or 10 large	1 fat
Pear, canned	½ c. or 2 halves	1 fruit
Pear with skin	½ large or 1 small	1 fruit
Peas (black-eyed, split), cooked	1 c.	2 bread + 1 lean meat
Peas (black-eyed, split), cooked	⅓ c.	1 bread
Peas, green	½ c.	1 bread
Pecans	2 large	1 fat
Peppers (all varieties)	^	FREE
Persimmon	2 medium	1 fruit
Picante sauce	^	FREE
Pickle relish	^	FREE
Pickles, unsweetened	^	FREE
Pimento	3 oz.	1 vegetable
Pimento loaf	1 oz.	1 meat + 1 fat
Pineapple, canned in own juice	⅓ c.	1 fruit
Pineapple juice	½ c.	1 fruit
Pineapple, raw	¾ c.	1 fruit
Pine nuts	1 tbsp.	1 fat
Pita	½ 6-in.	1 bread

* Foods with this symbol are high in saturated fat and are not recommended.
^ Daily total for FREE foods with this symbol should not exceed 50 calories.

Item	Amount	Exchanges
Plantain	½ c.	1 bread
Plums	2 small (5 oz.)	1 fruit
Pomegranate, raw	½ medium	1 fruit
Popcorn, air-popped, with no fat added	3 c.	1 bread
Pork chops	1 oz.	1 meat + ½ fat
Pork, high-fat (ground pork, pork sausage, spareribs)	1 oz.	1 meat + 1 fat
Pork, lean (boiled, canned, cured or fresh ham, Canadian bacon, tenderloin)	1 oz.	1 meat
Pork, medium-fat (Boston butts, chops, cutlets and loin roast)	1 oz.	1 meat + ½ fat
Pork sausage	1 oz.	1 meat + 1 fat
Potato, baked	1 small	1 bread
Potato, mashed	½ c.	1 bread
Potato, sweet, plain	⅓ c.	1 bread
Poultry (chicken with skin, domestic duck or goose, ground turkey)	1 oz.	1 meat + ½ fat
Poultry (Cornish game hen, skinless chicken, turkey)	1 oz.	1 meat
Pretzels	¾ oz.	1 bread
Prune juice	⅓ c.	1 fruit

* Foods with this symbol are high in saturated fat and are not recommended.
^ Daily total for FREE foods with this symbol should not exceed 50 calories.

Item	Amount	Exchanges
Prunes, dried	3 medium (1 oz.)	1 fruit
Pudding, sugar-free, prepared with fat-free milk	½ c.	½ milk + ½ bread
Puffed cereal (rice, wheat)	1½ c.	1 bread
Pumpkin, canned	¾ c.	1 bread
Pumpkin, home-cooked	¾ c.	½ bread
Pumpkin seeds	2 tsp.	1 fat
Radishes	1 c.	FREE
Raisin Bran Cereal	½ c.	1 bread
Raisin bread (unfrosted)	1 slice (1 oz.)	1 bread
Raisins	2 tbsp. (¼ oz.)	1 fruit
Raspberries	1 c.	1 fruit
Rhubarb, diced	2 c.	1 fruit
Rice (brown), cooked	½ c.	1 bread
Rice cakes	2 regular or 6 mini	1 bread
Rice Krispies	¾ c.	1 bread
Rice (white), cooked	⅓ c.	1 bread
Rice (wild), cooked	½ c.	1 bread
Ricotta cheese	¼ c.	1 meat + ½ fat
Roll, butter-style	1 small (1 oz.)	1 bread + 1 fat

R

* Foods with this symbol are high in saturated fat and are not recommended.
^ Daily total for FREE foods with this symbol should not exceed 50 calories.

Item	Amount	Exchanges
Roll, dinner	1 small (1 oz.)	1 bread
Romaine lettuce	1 c.	FREE
Rutabaga, raw	1 c.	1 vegetable
Rye Krisp	4 2x3½ in.	1 bread
S Salad dressing, fat-free	^	FREE
Salad dressing, light	1 tbsp.	1 fat
Salad dressing, regular	1 tsp.	1 fat
Salami	1 oz.	1 meat + 1 fat
Salsa	^	FREE
Salt pork	¼ oz.*	1 fat
Salt, seasoned	^	FREE
Sauerkraut	1 c.	1 vegetable
Sausage (Italian, pork, etc.)	1 oz.	1 meat + 1 fat
Shake, nutritional sugar-free (e.g., Alba Shake)	1 packet	1 milk
Shallots	4 tbsp.	1 vegetable
Shellfish (clams, crab, lobster, scallops, shrimp)	2 oz.	1 meat
Shortening	1 tsp.*	1 fat
Shredded wheat	½ c.	1 bread
Shrimp, fried	2 oz.	1 meat + 1 fat
Snow peas	½ c.	1 vegetable

* Foods with this symbol are high in saturated fat and are not recommended.
^ Daily total for FREE foods with this symbol should not exceed 50 calories.

Item	Amount	Exchanges
Soup, chicken noodle, canned	1 c.	½ bread + ½ fat
Soup, cream of broccoli, canned	½ c.	1 bread
Soup, cream of celery, canned	½ c.	1 bread
Soup, cream of chicken, canned	½ c.	1 bread + 1 fat
Soup, cream of mushroom, canned	½ c.	½ bread + 1 fat
Soup, vegetable beef, canned	1 c.	1 bread
Soup, vegetable, canned	1 c.	1 bread
Sour cream	2 tbsp.*	1 fat
Sour cream, fat-free	^	FREE
Sour cream, light	3 tbsp.*	1 fat
Soy sauce	^	FREE
Spareribs	1 oz.	1 meat + 1 fat
Spinach	1 c.	FREE
Spinach, cooked	½ c.	1 vegetable
Squash, cooked	¾ c.	1 bread
Steak sauce	^	FREE
Strawberries, frozen	1 c.	1 fruit
Strawberries, raw	1¼ c.	1 fruit
Stuffing, bread, prepared	¼ c.	1 bread + 1 fat
Sugar substitutes (all)	^	FREE

* Foods with this symbol are high in saturated fat and are not recommended.
^ Daily total for FREE foods with this symbol should not exceed 50 calories.

Item	Amount	Exchanges
Sunflower seeds, shelled	1 tbsp.	1 fat
Sweetbreads (high in cholesterol)	1 oz.	1 meat + ½ fat
Syrup, sugar-free	^	FREE
Tabasco sauce	^	FREE
Tabouli	2 tbsp.	1 bread + 1 fat
Taco sauce	^	FREE
Taco shell	1 6-in.	1 bread + 1 fat
Tangelos	1 medium	1 fruit
Tangerines	2 small (8 oz.)	1 fruit
Tapioca	2 tbsp.	1 bread
Tea (all types), unsweetened	^	FREE
Tempeh	½ c.	1 bread + 2 meats + 1 fat
Teriyaki sauce	^	FREE
Tofu	4 oz.	1 meat + ½ fat
Tomato	1 large	1 vegetable
Tomato juice	½ c.	1 vegetable
Tomato paste	6 tbsp.	1 bread
Tomato sauce	1 c.	1 bread
Tomato sauce (as condiment)	^	FREE

T

* Foods with this symbol are high in saturated fat and are not recommended.
^ Daily total for FREE foods with this symbol should not exceed 50 calories.

Item	Amount	Exchanges
Tonic water	^	FREE
Tortilla chips, baked	1 oz.	1 bread + 1 fat
Tortilla, corn	1 6-in.	1 bread
Tortilla, flour	1 6-in.	1 bread + 1 fat
Tuna, canned in oil	¼ c.	1 meat + ½ fat
Tuna, canned in water	¼ c.	1 meat
Turkey	1 oz.	1 meat
Turkey bacon	2 slices	1 meat + ½ fat
Turnips, cooked	½ c.	1 vegetable
Turnips, raw	1 c.	1 vegetable
Vanilla wafers, low-fat	8	1 bread + ½ fat
Veal, cutlet (ground or cubed, not breaded)	1 oz.	1 meat+ ½ fat
Veal, lean (all are lean except cutlets)	1 oz. ground or cubed	1 meat
Vegetable beef soup, canned	1 c.	1 bread
Vegetable juice	½ c.	1 vegetable
Vegetable soup, canned	1 c.	1 bread
Vinegar (all types)	^	FREE

V

* Foods with this symbol are high in saturated fat and are not recommended.
^ Daily total for FREE foods with this symbol should not exceed 50 calories.

	Item	Amount	Exchanges
W	Waffle (5x5x½ inch)	1	1 bread + 1 fat
	Walnuts	2 whole	1 fat
	Water chestnuts	½ c.	1 vegetable
	Watercress	1 c.	FREE
	Watermelon cubes	1¼ c.	1 fruit
	Wheat germ	3 tbsp.	1 bread
	Wheat germ (toasted)	¼ c.	1 bread + 1 lean meat
	Wheaties	¾ c.	1 bread
	Whipped topping	3 tbsp.*	1 fat
	Whipped topping, fat-free	^	FREE
	Whipping cream	1 tbsp.*	1 fat
	Worcestershire sauce	^	FREE
Y	Yam, sweet potato, plain	⅓ c.	1 bread
	Yogurt, fat-free and sugar-free	8 oz.	1 milk
	Yogurt, frozen, nonfat	3 oz.	1 bread
	Yogurt, low-fat sugar-free	8 oz.	1 milk + 1 fat
	Yogurt, plain sugar-free	8 oz.	1 milk + 2 fats
Z	Zucchini, cooked	½ c.	1 vegetable
	Zucchini, raw	1 c.	FREE

* Foods with this symbol are high in saturated fat and are not recommended.
^ Daily total for FREE foods with this symbol should not exceed 50 calories.

FAST-FOOD RESTAURANT HEALTHY CHOICES

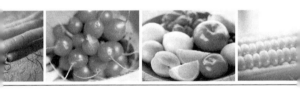

Item	Exchanges
Arby's (www.arbys.com)	
Arby's Sauce (1 pkg.)	FREE
Au jus sauce (1 pkg.)	FREE
Baked potato (plain)	5 breads
Homestyle French fries (small)	2 breads, 2 fats
Garden salad (no dressing)	2 vegetables
Grilled chicken BBQ sandwich	$2\frac{1}{2}$ meats, 3 breads, 1 fat
Hot ham and Swiss sandwich	3 meats, 2 breads, $1\frac{1}{2}$ fats
Light roast chicken deluxe sandwich	2 meats, 2 breads
Light roast turkey deluxe sandwich	2 meats, 2 breads
Reduced-calorie buttermilk ranch dressing (1 pkg.)	1 bread
Reduced-calorie Italian dressing (1 pkg.)	FREE
Regular roast beef sandwich	3 meats, 2 breads, $1\frac{1}{2}$ fats
Roast chicken salad (no dressing)	3 meats, 2 vegetables
Super roast beef sandwich	3 meats, 3 breads, $3\frac{1}{2}$ fats

Item	Exchanges
Baja Fresh Mexican Grill (www.bajafresh.com)	
Baja Burrito with chicken	4 meats, 3 breads, 5 fats
Baja Burrito with chicken (no cheese)	4 meats, 3 breads, 2 fats
Baja Burrito with steak (no cheese)	$3\frac{1}{2}$ meats, 3 breads, 3 fats
Baja fish taco	1 meat, 1 bread, 1 fat
Burrito Mexicano with chicken	4 meats, 6 breads, $1\frac{1}{2}$ fats
Burrito Mexicano with steak	4 meats, 6 breads, $2\frac{1}{2}$ fats
Fresh charbroiled fish taco (with Mahi Mahi)	$1\frac{1}{2}$ meats, 1 bread, $1\frac{1}{2}$ fats
Mini Quesa-Dita	2 meats, $4\frac{1}{2}$ breads, 2 fats
Mini Quesa-Dita with steak	3 meats, $4\frac{1}{2}$ breads, 2 fats
Original Baja Style Taco with chicken	1 meat, 1 bread
Original Baja Style Taco with shrimp	1 meat, 1 bread
Original Baja Style Taco with steak	1 meat, 1 bread
Taco Chilito with chicken	2 meats, 2 breads, 2 fats
Taco Chilito with chicken (no cheese/sour cream)	2 meats, 2 breads

Item	Exchanges
Taco Chilito with steak	2 meats, 2 breads, 2 fats
Taco Chilito with steak (no cheese/sour cream)	2 meats, 2 breads
Torta with steak	3 meats, $3\frac{1}{2}$ breads, 8 fats
Torta with steak (no mayonnaise/sour cream)	3 meats, $3\frac{1}{2}$ breads, 2 fats
Torta with chicken	3 meats, $3\frac{1}{2}$ breads, 7 fats
Torta with chicken (no mayonnaise/sour cream)	3 meats, $3\frac{1}{2}$ breads, 1 fat
Tortilla chips (15 chips)	1 bread, $1\frac{1}{2}$ fats

Item	Exchanges

Burger King (www.burgerking.com)

Item	Exchanges
BK Broiler with chicken (no sauce)	3 meats, 3 breads, 1 fat
Chicken Caesar salad (no dressing/croutons)	3 meats, 2 vegetables
Chicken Tenders (8 pieces)	3 meats, 1 bread, 1½ fats
Fat-free Italian dressing (1 pkg.)	FREE
Garden salad (no dressing)	½ meat, 1 vegetable, 1 fat
Hamburger	2 meats, 2 breads, 2 fats
Minute Maid orange juice	2 fruits

Carl's Jr. (www.carlsjr.com)

Item	Exchanges
Baked Potato (plain)	4 breads
Big Burger	3 meats, 3 breads, 1½ fats
Breadsticks (1 pkg.)	½ bread
Breakfast quesadilla	2 meats, 2 breads, 1 fat
Charbroiled BBQ chicken sandwich	4 meats, 2 breads
Charbroiled chicken Salad-to-go	3½ meats, 2 vegetables
Chicken Stars (6 pieces)	1½ meats, 1 bread, 1½ fats

Item	Exchanges
Fat-free French dressing (1 pkg.)	1 bread
Fat-free Italian dressing (1 pkg.)	FREE
French fries (small)	3 breads, 3 fats
Hamburger	1 meat, 1½ breads, ½ fat

Chick-fil-A (www.chickfila.com)

Item	Exchanges
Carrot and raisin salad (small)	2 vegetables, 1 fruit
Chick-fil-A Chargrilled Chicken Deluxe Sandwich	3 meats, 2 breads
Chick-fil-A Chargrilled Chicken Garden Salad	4 lean meats, 1 vegetable
Chick-fil-A Chick-N-Strips (4 pieces)	4 meats, 1 bread
Chick-fil-A Chick-N-Strips Salad	4½ meats, 1 bread, 1 fat
Chick-fil-A Chicken Sandwich	3 meats, 2½ breads, 1 fat
Chick-fil-A Waffle Potato Fries (small)	3 breads, 2 fats
Chicken salad plate	3 meats, 2 breads
Diet lemonade	FREE
Hearty breast of chicken soup (single serving)	1 lean meat, ½ bread
IceDream (small cone)	1 bread, 1 fat

Item	Exchanges

Dairy Queen (www.dairyqueen.com)

Item	Exchanges
Chicken breast fillet sandwich	3 meats, 2½ breads, 1½ fats
DQ fudge bar (no sugar added)	1 bread
DQ Homestyle hamburger	2 meats, 2 breads, 1 fat
DQ vanilla-orange bar (no sugar added)	1 bread
Grilled chicken sandwich	3 meats, 2 breads

Domino's (www.dominos.com)

Item	Exchanges
Large Classic hand-tossed cheese pizza (2 slices)	1 meat, 3 breads, 1½ fats
Large Crunchy thin-crust cheese pizza (2 slices)	1 meat, 2 breads, 1½ fats
Side salad (with 2 tbsp. fat-free dressing)	1 vegetable
Toppings (ham, vegetables, pineapple, per slice)	FREE

Item	Exchanges
Hardees (www.hardees.com)	
Apple Cinnamon 'N' Raisin biscuit	2 breads, 1 fat
Baked beans (small)	2 breads
Chicken fillet sandwich	3 meats, $3\frac{1}{2}$ breads, $1\frac{1}{2}$ fats
Fat-free French dressing (1 pkg.)	FREE
French fries (small)	2 breads, 2 fats
Grilled chicken salad (no dressing)	3 meats, 2 vegetables
Grilled chicken sandwich	3 meats, $2\frac{1}{2}$ breads
Hamburger	2 meats, 2 breads, 1 fat
Hot Ham 'N' Cheese	2 meats, 1 bread, 1 fat
Ice-cream cone	2 breads
Mashed potatoes (small)	1 bread
Orange juice	2 fruits
Side salad (no dressing)	1 vegetable

Item	Exchanges
Jack In the Box (www.jackinthebox.com)	
Breakfast Jack	2 meats, 2 breads, 1 fat
Chicken breast pieces (5 pieces)	3 meats, 1½ breads, 2 fats
Chicken fajita pita	3 meats, 1½ breads
Garden chicken salad	3 meats, 1 vegetable
Hamburger	1½ meats, 2 breads, ¾ fat
Low-calorie Italian dressing (1 pkg.)	FREE
Side salad (no dressing)	1 vegetable
KFC (www.kfc.com)	
BBQ baked beans	2 breads, ½ fat
Coleslaw	1 bread, 1 vegetable, 2 fats
Colonel's Crispy Strips (3 pieces)	3 meats, ½ bread, 1½ fats
Corn-on-the-cob (1 ear)	2 breads, ½ fat
Honey BBQ flavored chicken sandwich	2 meats, 2 breads
Hot and spicy drumstick	2 meats, ½ breads, 1 fat
Garden rice (single serving)	1½ breads
Green beans (single serving)	1 vegetable

Item	Exchanges
Macaroni and cheese (single serving)	1½ breads, 1 fat
Mashed potatoes with gravy (single serving)	1 bread, 1 fat
Original Recipe drumstick	2 meats, ½ breads, 1 fat
Tender Roast breast (no skin)	4½ meats
Tender Roast drumstick (no skin)	1½ meats
Tender Roast thigh (no skin)	2 lean meats

Little Caesar's (www.littlecaesars.com)

Item	Exchanges
Caesar salad (no dressing)	1 meat, 3 vegetables, ½ fat
Crazy Bread (1 slice)	1 bread, ½ fat
Crazy Sauce (4 oz.)	1 bread
Fat-free Italian dressing (1 pkg.)	FREE
Medium (14-in.) Pan! Pan! cheese pizza (1 slice)	1 meat, 1½ breads, ½ fat
Medium (14-in.) Pan! Pan! pepperoni pizza (1 slice)	1 meat, 1½ breads, 1 fat
Tossed salad (no dressing)	3 vegetables, ½ fat

Item	Exchanges

Long John Silver's (www.longjohnsilvers.com)

Item	Exchanges
Baked potato (plain)	3 breads
Batter-dipped fish sandwich (no sauce)	2 meats, 2 breads, 1 fat
Cole slaw	1 bread, 1 fat
Corn cobbette (no butter)	1 bread
FlavorBaked chicken (no sauce)	2½ meats
FlavorBaked fish	2 meats
FlavorBaked chicken sandwich (no sauce)	2½ meats, 2 breads
Green beans (single serving)	1 vegetable
Rice pilaf	2 breads
Side salad (no dressing)	1 vegetable

McDonald's (www.mcdonalds.com)

Item	Exchanges
Chicken McGrill (plain)	3 meats, 2½ breads
Egg McMuffin	2 meats, 2 breads, 1 fat
English muffin	2 breads
Garden salad (no dressing)	1 vegetable
Grilled chicken Caesar salad (no dressing)	3 meats, 1 vegetable
Fat-free herb vinaigrette dressing (1 pkg.)	½ bread

Item	Exchanges
Hamburger	1½ meats, 2 breads, ¾ fat
Hash browns	1 bread, 1 fat
Honey mustard dressing (1 pkg.)	1 bread, 2 fats
Hotcakes (plain)	3½ breads, 1 fat
Low-fat ice-cream cone	½ bread, ½ milk, 1 fat
McSalad Shaker chef salad (no dressing)	2½ lean meats, 1 vegetable
McSalad Shaker garden salad (no dressing)	1 medium-fat meat, 1 vegetable
McSalad Shaker grilled chicken Caesar salad (no dressing)	1½ very lean meats, 1 vegetable
Orange juice	2 fruits
Quarter Pounder	3 meats, 2½ breads, 1½ fats
Ranch dressing (1 pkg.)	4 fats
Reduced-fat Red French dressing (1 pkg.)	1 bread, 1 fat
Scrambled eggs (2)	2 meats, 1 fat
Thousand Island dressing (1 pkg.)	1 bread, 2 fats

Item	Exchanges
Pizza Hut (www.pizzahut.com)	
Hand-tossed cheese pizza (1 slice)	2 meats, 2 breads, 1 fat
Thin 'n Crispy cheese pizza (1 slice)	1 meat, 1½ breads, 1½ fats
Veggie Lover's Thin 'n Crispy pizza (1 slice)	1 meat, 1½ breads, ½ fat
Veggie Lover's hand-tossed pizza (1 slice)	1 meat, 2 breads, ½ fat
Rubio's Fresh Mexican Grill (www.rubios.com)	
Beans (side serving)	1 meat, 2 breads
Beans and rice (side serving)	1 meat, 6 breads, 1½ fats
Carne asada taco	1½ meats, 1½ breads, 1 fat
Cheese quesadilla	2 meats, 2½ breads, 4½ fats
Fish taco	1 meat, 2 breads, 2 fats
Fish taco especial	1½ meats, 2 breads, 3 fats
Grilled chicken taco	2 meats, 1½ breads, 2 fats
Grilled fish taco	2 meats, 1½ breads, 2 fats

Item	Exchanges
Grilled Grande Bowl with chicken	2 meats, 5 breads
Grilled Grande Bowl with carne asada	2 meats, 5 breads, ½ fat
Guacamole (small)	3½ fats
HealthMex chicken burrito	3 meats, 4 breads, 1 fat
HealthMex chicken taco	1½ meats, 1 bread
HealthMex grilled fish burrito	3 meats, 4 breads, ½ fat
HealthMex grilled fish taco	1½ meats, 1 bread
Rice (side order)	3 breads, ½ fat
Rice (side serving with HealthMex entrée)	1½ breads
Salsa (all types)	FREE
Taquitos (3)	2 meats, 1½ breads, 2 fats
Tortilla chips (side order)	3½ breads, 5½ fats
Tortilla chips (side serving with burrito)	1½ breads, 2 fats

Item	Exchanges
Subway (www.subway.com)	
7 Under 6 ham salad (no dressing)	1 meat, 2 vegetables
7 Under 6 ham sandwich (6-in.)	2 meats, 3 breads
7 Under 6 roast beef salad (no dressing)	1 meat, 2 vegetables
7 Under 6 roast beef sandwich (6-in.)	2 meats, 3 breads
7 Under 6 roasted chicken breast salad (no dressing)	1 meat, 3 vegetables
7 Under 6 roasted chicken breast sandwich (6-in.)	3 meats, 3 breads
7 Under 6 Subway Club salad (no dressing)	2 meats, 2 vegetables
7 Under 6 turkey breast and ham salad (no dressing)	1 meat, 2 vegetables
7 Under 6 turkey breast sandwich (6-in.)	2 meats, 3 breads
7 Under 6 Veggie Delite sandwich (6-in.)	3 breads
Cold Cut Trio sandwich (6-in.)	2 meats, 3 breads, 1 fat
Fat-free French dressing (1 pkg.)	FREE
Fat-free Italian dressing (1 pkg.)	FREE
Meatball sandwich (6-in.)	2 meats, $3\frac{1}{2}$ breads, 1 fat
Steak and cheese sandwich (6-in.)	3 meats, 3 breads
Subway melt sandwich (6-in.)	2 meats, 3 breads, 1 fat

Item	Exchanges
Taco Bell (www.tacobell.com)	
Bean burrito	1 meat, 3 breads, 1½ fats
Chicken soft taco	1½ meats, 1½ breads
Pintos and cheese	1 meat, ½ bread, 1½ fats
Steak soft taco	2 meats, 1 bread
TCBY (www.tcby.com)	
Nonfat frozen yogurt (½ c.)	1½ breads
No-sugar added, nonfat frozen yogurt (½ c.)	1 bread

Item	Exchanges
Wendy's (www.wendys.com)	
Baked potato (with sour cream and chives)	4½ breads, 1 fat
Baked potato (plain)	4 breads
Caesar side salad (no dressing)	1 meat, 1 vegetable, ½ fat
Chili (small)	2 meats, 1 bread, 1 fat
Fat-free Italian dressing (1 pkg.)	FREE
Garden ranch chicken pita	4 meats, 3 breads
Grilled chicken salad (no dressing)	3 meats, 2 vegetables
Grilled chicken sandwich	3 meats, 2 breads
Junior hamburger	1 meat, 2 breads, ½ fat
Side salad (no dressing)	1 vegetable
Wendy's single hamburger (plain)	3 meats, 2 breads, 1½ fats

GREAT FIRST PLACE BOOKS TO HELP YOU TRANSFORM YOUR LIFE IN EVERY WAY!

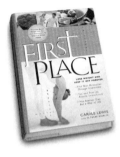

This introduction to the nation's leading Christian weight-loss program shows you how to lose weight, keep it off and strengthen your body and soul!

First Place
Carole Lewis with *Terry Whalin*
Hardcover • ISBN 08307.28635

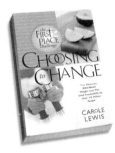

Carole Lewis tells how First Place became the nation's number one Christian weight-loss program and explains the nine commitments that are the program's central focus.

Choosing to Change
Carole Lewis
Paperback • ISBN 08307.28627

HERE'S ALL YOU NEED TO START A FIRST PLACE GROUP AT YOUR CHURCH!

Group Starter Kit
ISBN 08307.28708

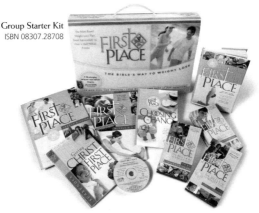

The **First Place Group Starter Kit** includes *Leader's Guide*, *Member's Guide*, *Giving Christ First Place* Bible Study with Scripture Memory Music CD, *First Place* and *Choosing to Change* books and four videos—*Nine Commitments*, *Orientation*, *Food Exchange Plan* and *An Introduction to First Place*.

EVERY FIRST PLACE MEMBER NEEDS A MEMBER'S KIT AND A FIRST PLACE BIBLE STUDY!

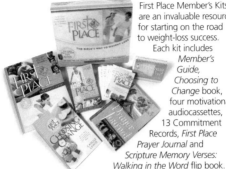

First Place Member's Kits are an invaluable resource for starting on the road to weight-loss success. Each kit includes *Member's Guide, Choosing to Change* book, four motivational audiocassettes, 13 Commitment Records, *First Place Prayer Journal* and *Scripture Memory Verses: Walking in the Word* flip book.

Member's Kit • ISBN 08307.28708

Choose from These Life-Changing Bible Studies — Each with a Scripture Memory Music CD!

Giving Christ First Place • ISBN 08307.28643
Everyday Victory for Everyday People • ISBN 08307.28651
Life Under Control • ISBN 08307.29305
Life That Wins • ISBN 08307.29240
Seeking God's Best • ISBN 08307.29259
Pressing On to the Prize • ISBN 08307.29267
Pathway to Success • ISBN 08307.29275
Living the Legacy • ISBN 08307.29283
Making Wise Choices • ISBN 08307.30818
Begin Again • ISBN 08307.32330

Pick up First Place Member's Kits and Bible Studies where Christian books are sold!

www.firstplace.org

Gospel Light

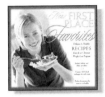
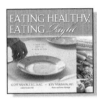